Suburban Survival Guide

How to Break the Sugar Habit in Your Family

Jay Foard

ISBN: 098987432X
ISBN-13: 9780989874328
Library of Congress Control Number: 2013915444
LCCN Imprint Name: CVFPublishing, Ponte Vedra,
Florida

To Fiorella, Connor, and Tyler

My inspiration to want what is best for all families

Note on References

For my previous book, I spent a lot of time referencing information and documenting sources. For this book, I've decided to skip this for the most part and save the trees. My primary objective isn't to convince the reader of specific quantitative facts and figures. These are available from an online search, and readers can do what I have done and research the information as necessary for any area they may not agree with or want to dispute.

From my perspective, it isn't important, for instance, if a trend is rising precisely 35.7 percent or 45.2 percent year over year. There are always assumptions and parameters associated with these statistics, and it can be difficult to have apples-to-apples comparisons, given different approaches to the numbers. This book is focused on the qualitative position that the rise in trends such as type 2 juvenile diabetes is substantial, and something needs to be done to protect our children from the devastating consequences it has on them. It is more about strategy and less about getting bogged down by numbers and conflicting scientific research studies. I have made every effort to research the topic by filtering the information in a way that I think makes it easier to understand without compromising on the science behind it.

Note on Terminology

There are two types of diabetes (type 1 and type 2), which can be confusing. Type 1 diabetes is a chronic condition with a strong genetic component in which the pancreas produces little or no insulin. It used to be termed "juvenile diabetes" because it typically occurs early in life. This terminology has now changed because type 2 diabetes is becoming more prevalent in children and young adults. Type 2 diabetes is typically associated with insulin resistance and influenced by lifestyle habits. Because of this, the focus is on type 2 diabetes and the factors we can control through diet, exercise, and interaction with our environment.

Defining the word *sugar* can itself be a difficult discussion. Sugar is a type of carbohydrate, and depending on its chemical composition, it comes in many forms and variations. Carbohydrates are measured in units of weight but are usually thought about in units of heat energy, called calories, needed to raise temperature.

There are simple sugars, called monosaccharides, that make up many of the sugars we are familiar with, such as glucose and fructose. There are starches and complex sugars, called polysaccharides, that are long chains of connected sugar compounds. Some sugars are digested and absorbed into the bloodstream very quickly, while others need to be broken down in the digestive process and take longer to enter the bloodstream. This, along with other factors, plays a part in how the sugar affects health. Simple carbohydrates that are digested quickly tend to increase insulin levels faster, which is an important factor in how your body is managing the sugar intake.

Nutritionists, dietitians, and health practitioners take many factors related to carbohydrates into consideration when they develop a holistic health strategy. The point of this book is to keep the topic simple. I'm aiming to avoid the confusion and scientific jargon while still being factual and results based. I use the term *sugar* in very general terms because, although it matters when developing a nutritional plan, I don't think the readers have to be concerned whether they are consuming a monosaccharide or polysaccharide in order to better understand how sugar is affecting the health of their families and what can be done about it at the consumer level.

This book is intended to bring awareness and new thought on the subject, and I encourage readers to consult with a professional health practitioner about dietary adjustments if they're serious about making changes to their eating habits and lifestyles.

Contents

Preface

As a parent, I understand clearly the challenges in today's society when it comes to our children's health. We all want what is best for our children, but unfortunately in the United States, where I live, along with many other countries, we have some of the unhealthiest children in the world. That seems to defy reason. What is going on? In this book I will explore the topic and, I hope, help parents develop a new outlook on health and learn what they can do differently for their families.

I'm going to embark on a tangent because it is important for parents to understand the types of challenges they are up against when trying to find a sustainable approach to keeping their children healthy. We live in a society that is measured by corporate growth. This corporate growth feeds into economic growth, which provides the jobs we need to sustain our families. From that perspective we are glad to have jobs and need to have a stable, growing economy.

One of the challenges with this is that corporate growth is based on consumer consumption. Success is measured by how well a company can convince consumers (namely, us and our families) to purchase its goods and services. With high levels of competition and quarterly sales expectations, corporations will go to extremes to sell their products. They also are willing to compromise on quality if they can reach sales targets and exceed profit margins by using cheaper commodity ingredients or clever marketing campaigns.

It's not surprising that marketing departments spend a lot of money to understand consumer behavior and how to sell products. They have done a great job of distilling the data about what consumers are most likely to consume or purchase down to their core psychological and physiological cravings. This has given rise to what I call the three Ss of marketing used by companies to sell the largest majority of consumable goods: sugar, salt, and sex (not necessarily in that order).

This does not mean that sugar and salt are the only ingredients that are unhealthful in food products. They are just used as base ingredients to market and sell goods, many of which have lots of other unhealthful ingredients as well, such as fats, artificial flavors, modified chemicals, residuals from pesticides sprayed on foods, and other ingredients we do not want our children to consume. The other bad ingredients are also detrimental to health and affect our children in many ways.

For this book, I'm focusing on sugar and sometimes salt, because cutting down on sugar and salt usually means cutting down on all those other bad ingredients as well. I'll leave the sex aspect for a different book by a different author!

Another challenge is that while companies measure the result of their inputs, they are not usually concerned with the outputs. For example, a soft drink or cupcake company would love to have you and your family consume their products all day every day. This is great for the company's quarterly profits and corporate growth. But what if the products are bad for the consumer? What if they are linked to obesity or diabetes or other long-term health conditions? What level of responsibility do companies that overmarket their products to the point of overconsumption have when it comes to the result of their outputs?

When I was doing my graduate work at the Duke Business School, someone from a large consumer goods company came in to talk about its growth strategy into new markets. The company was extremely excited (and proud of itself) for coming up with new ways to penetrate tribal rural areas of India and Latin America to distribute their packaged goods, mostly in small single-package amounts such as single-wash laundry soap or bar soaps. They did this by setting up small businesses that leveraged women in the communities and paying them small fees for selling their products. It was a clever approach to driving more sales into a hard-to-reach consumer base. The women made a small profit as entrepreneurs within the tribe.

But I have a background in biology, and I've visited many of these rural areas. Something bothered me. In the past, these tribal areas made their own supplies by hand out of available natural resources, and they were biodegradable. This new era of packaged goods created

3

an output problem because the packages were nonbiodegradable, making them difficult to dispose of. Companies work exceptionally hard to get their goods to these hard-to-reach places, but what about the thousands of little plastic packages and wrappers that are leftover?

In the United States, there is typically a sophisticated garbage pickup and recycling service, and most Americans just leave their plastic wrappers and packages in garbage bags by the street to be carried away. In rural villages, however, there is usually no infrastructure or service like this available. The plastic packages flow over in garbage cans and litter streets. I remember seeing a desert in South America that was strewn with thousands of plastic bags and containers that had blown across from the neighboring pueblos. I've seen people in India dumping trash cans full of plastic containers and other garbage over seawalls.

During this presentation I went so far as to ask, "After working so hard and spending so much money to convince consumers in these rural areas to buy your products, do you do anything to help remove the empty wrappers, bottles, cans, and packages that are left behind?" I did not get a good answer.

Corporations focus on funding the front-end sales cycle and promoting consumption. They are not fond of spending money to fund cleanup activities as a result of consumer purchases unless they are forced to by some sort of government or advocate policy or as the result of a catastrophe. When we think about what we are inputting, we have to consider the consequences of the outputs. Overconsumption often becomes someone else's problem. In reality it becomes the consumers' problem.

Our bodies face the same problem as these rural villages. Part of anything we input has to be disposed of through an output. We can use some of what we consume. In the villages consumers can use the actual laundry detergent to clean their clothes. But we do not use some of it, such as the plastic wrappers, and those have to be disposed of or stored, which can be difficult. The output of plastic containers turns into litter that pollutes the streets of villages and builds up. The output of unhealthy food turns into litter that pollutes our bodies and deprecates our health.

If we take this example and extend it to the consumer level, what sorts of problems does overconsumption cause our families? Do we see the impact on our children in terms of their health and wellness? Based on the health trends in the United States, the resulting output has gotten to the point of becoming a catastrophe.

Let's take this a step further to understand how these inputs and outputs pertain to disease. We know that genetic inheritance plays an important role in our overall health and well-being. We also know that our environment plays an important role in our health. How do we determine what we can control through our environment versus what we inherit?

In my previous book, *Run Your Body Like a Business*, I use a business analogy to explain this, referencing the concept of alpha/beta factors to describe DNA versus environmental influence. That book was written for readers with a business background, but let's look at this a different way.

Say you're going to bake a cake based on a recipe you *inherited* from a chef. How well the cake turns out directly depends on how well you follow the recipe, with the ingredients and your environment working together as inputs. The recipe and ingredients play an important role. Some ingredients are used in larger quantities and others in smaller quantities, even though they are just as important.

If we change the recipe, how much does that change the resulting cake? Some changes may be subtle. Leaving out a teaspoonful of flour may not even be noticeable. Other changes to the ingredients can have a big impact. Adding five eggs instead of two completely changes the texture of the cake. Different ingredients serve different purposes. A teaspoonful of vanilla extract helps the taste. A teaspoonful of baking soda affects the chemistry as the cake is baking.

Environmental factors that you control also play a significant role. You can take two cakes with the same ingredients but have a very different result by changing an environmental factor, like the cooking time. How would your cake turn out if you cooked it at 375° F for ten minutes versus one hour versus six hours?

The body works in the same way. Genes basically use a recipe that instructs each cell on how to make more cells. Different cells have different active genes (recipes), which is how liver cells know how to make more liver cells and skin cells know how to make more skin cells. All of the cells use environmental inputs as ingredients. Sometimes this works for us and sometimes against us. Skin cells, for instance, get vitamin D from the sun, which is beneficial to the health of the cell. They can also get UV radiation from the sun, which can be dangerous and lead to skin cancer, especially if there is a genetic disposition already. Our genes' recipes and environment inputs affect the health of individual cells that when aggregated together are the organs and systems that give us life.

Unfortunately, some children are born with genetic predispositions (the recipe is essentially incorrect) that cause congenital illnesses or make them more susceptible to certain types of early childhood diseases, which can affect their health in sometimes tragic ways, despite their environment. The most prevalent increases in disease, however, can be tied back to how we are interacting with our environment. If children have significant overconsumption of toxic substances (i.e., sugar) at an early age, then by the time they reach their teens or twenties, they have had potentially years of abuse. This is a contributing factor to the soaring rates of type 2 juvenile diabetes.

One study, for instance, found that "People who

7

consume sugary drinks regularly—one to two cans a day or more—have a 26 percent greater risk of developing type 2 diabetes than people who rarely have such drinks." This study is only looking at *soft drink consumption.* Imagine what the percentage is when we factor in all the other sugary products our children consume on a regular basis. We'll discuss this in more detail shortly.

To think about health for our families holistically, we need to consider the different inputs and how those affect our outputs. This book is to help empower parents to better understand how inputs might be affecting their children's health and provide ideas on what they can do to have better health strategies for their families.

As I mentioned before, there are many aspects of diet that affect a child's health, including damage from fried foods and saturated oils and carcinogens from chemicals in pesticides. Although these factors are a major consideration, one key ingredient proven to be detrimental to a child's long-term health that is ubiquitous in all these products is one I call the invited assassin.

The Invited Assassin

Children do not come with a manual. It can be a tricky business figuring out how to handle different types of threats to our children. Here in Florida, there are a lot of parents scared to let their children play in the yard or around bodies of water because of snakes and alligators. Many parents fear that their children will get sick if they are wet or out in the rain (even though being wet and/or cold is rarely a contributing factor to contracting an illness, disease, or infection, which is caused by contact with a bacterium or virus). Parents of teenagers worry about sex, cigarettes, alcohol, drugs, and peer pressure. It is built into our biology to go to any extreme to protect our children from threats or danger.

But here is an irony. One of the most dangerous threats to our children in today's suburban lifestyle comes from something we not only welcome into our homes but actually pay for, and our children consume it on a regular basis. It's more dangerous than almost any other threat that keeps parents up at night. What is this? It is the overconsumption of sugar from the foods they are eating.

I already anticipate the reader's cynicism. Surely I'm exaggerating. Given how prevalent these foods have become in our society and daily routine, consuming them is just normal. In a minute I'm going to explain why overconsumption of sugar is such a threat, and what has changed so dramatically, but first let's talk about this concept of normal.

Normal is a funny thing. Routines, habits, and influences seep into our lives and become embedded. Before we realize it, what we consider normal is not normal at all. Childhood obesity is not normal. In fact, children having excess fat or being chubby is not usually normal in terms of how the body works. This comment may cause controversy with some parents and practitioners who point out that bodies work differently and some children have a genetic disposition to being overweight which I acknowledge throughout the book. My point is that for most children excess weight can be attributed to poor diet. Having excess body fat from poor diet works against the health of the child and against how the body functions. It causes unnecessary strain on the heart and other organs and systems, for instance, along with many health-related factors that could be avoided simply through diet.

We fall into all sorts of traps when it comes to what we consider normal. Turning on the news in major US cities and hearing headlines about murder and shootings should not be considered normal, although we have come to accept it in today's world. But that is also a book for another day.

With regard to food consumption, we tend to fall into the herd mentality when it comes to clever marketing, and we ignore the real indicators. Overweight children are typically overconsuming the wrong foods. Plain and simple.

There are all sorts of contradictory studies on foods and their impact on health as it relates to children, most of which are noise and muddle the topic. At the Harvard University School of Public Health website (https://www.hsph.harvard.edu/nutritionsource/sugary -drinks-fact-sheet/), for instance, you can find the following information:

- Beverage companies in the United States spent roughly $3.2 billion marketing carbonated beverages in 2006, with nearly a half-billion dollars of that marketing aimed directly at youth ages 2–17.
- And each year, youth see hundreds of television ads for sugar-containing drinks. In 2010, for example, preschoolers viewed an average of 213 ads for sugary drinks and energy drinks, while children and teens watched an average of 277 and 406 ads, respectively.
- Yet the beverage industry aggressively rebuffs suggestions that its products and marketing tactics play any role in the obesity epidemic.
- Adding to the confusion, beverage industry-funded studies are four to eight times more likely to show a finding favorable to industry than independently funded studies.

The simple fact is children today in the United States and many countries overconsume carbohydrates in the form of sugar. Sugar is the staple ingredient that sells almost all goods aimed at children, so it is in the interest of producers to muddle the topic. What makes the problem of overconsumption of sugar so dangerous is that the damage is done over time. Products consumed today and tomorrow may not seem to be causing an immediate impact on our children's health (besides obesity, laziness, disciplinary, and self-esteem problems). But what happens over time is what matters. Sometimes over a decade or longer.

As parents, we understand the importance in investing in our children's future. We know, for instance, we should start saving early for college tuition, and, if possible, we set up funds while they are in elementary school to pay for college later. This is a good investment. With consistent sugar consumption, we are making a bad long-term investment in our children's health. Why does our logic become so turned around?

To better explain, let's use a simple analogy. Say when your child was born, $5 million was also included that the child can have when he or she turns eighteen. What do you do with that money as a parent for eighteen years while the child is under your guidance? Surely as the parent you would save the money, right? Would you be willing to pull amounts out all along for the child just because he or she jumps up and down and begs to buy frivolous and transitory items? How often and how much would you spend? Some of it? All of it?

What do children do once they are grown up and can make their own decisions? They may decide to squander the money, but at least as the parent you did your part helping preserve the money and leaving them in a good financial position. But if you participate in helping them squander it, what happens when they get to eighteen and there is none left?

Now let's apply the same logic to health. When we have a child, we only hope it is a healthy baby. Essentially hoping the child has those five million "life dollars" in the bank. Unfortunately, in the game of life, we don't know how many life dollars we'll start with. That is determined by our genes. We do know that every time we do something that compromises our health, we are losing life dollars a bit at a time. Take, for example, cigarette smoking. As part of the Cancer Genome Project, it was found that a lung cancer cell has "approximately 23,000 individual mutations." This means that a typical smoker develops one mutation for every fifteen cigarettes he or she smokes. Every puff of a cigarette is costing life dollars, handfuls at a time.

Even though it is less obvious, overconsumption of sugar has the same impact as cigarette smoking over time. (I know there are some parents who choke at such a comparison, but I'll discuss the parallels soon.) Researchers don't know the full effect, and there are a lot of factors at play. But if you let your child start eating sugary foods at two years old, and let a child eat too much sugar for eighteen years, how much is left in the bank at thirty? Or more to the point, how much damage has been done? Once your children are adults and can make their own decisions, how many life dollars did you leave for them? If you were smart and didn't squander their life dollars, are they as smart about their health as they should be about money, able to make good decisions on their own in the future?

Some of the damage can be offset. If you are consuming high amounts of sugar but also eating other healthy items and getting exercise, you are probably putting money back in the bank. You typically do not know whether it is enough to counter the damage until later in life. One challenge is how do toddlers, who can barely walk, get enough exercise to offset adult portions of sugar in cookies, cupcakes, pudding, ice cream, and all of the other high-concentration sugar items many tend to eat on a regular basis? Too often parents give these concentrated sugar products to children who aren't even old enough to be out of a high chair, so they can post pictures of their baby's face covered in cupcake icing on Facebook. How much life money is it costing, based on damage to organs that have not even fully formed yet along with other important systems such as the endocrine and central nervous systems? How does it affect a heart that is only the size of their fist?

This may seem abstract, but it is supported by research and seen in the current epidemic of type 2 juvenile diabetes in young adults (yesterday's children). If we were not compromising our children's health with high sugar intake early in life, along with lack of exercise, those rates would not be increasing. Unfortunately, not only are they increasing; they are skyrocketing here in the United States and many other countries.

To put this in perspective, consider that the diagnosed cases of diabetes in the United States have increased by 382 percent from 1988 to 2014. (Wouldn't we have loved our stock portfolios to have this type of increase?) The sad part is diabetes is a systemic disease, which means it manifests with all sorts of residual health implications, including heart attacks, strokes, blindness, amputation, and kidney disease.

Sugar is also a contributing factor to increasing cancer rates, primarily in adults because, as with type 2 diabetes, the damage is done over time. Sugar is the fuel that feeds cancer cells, as it does all cells. Cancer cells fundamentally work by producing proteins that stimulate blood vessel formation to redirect the supply of nutrients, including sugar, so the tumor can grow and proliferate. Research studies have demonstrated a direct link between type 2 diabetes (insulin resistance) and cancer.

I believe that overconsumption of sugar is on a par with cigarette smoking when it comes to our children's health. Sugar is the new nicotine. I understand when parents are skeptical of this comparison. On the surface it should make sense. Both smoking and high sugar consumption affect health systemically over time and are similar to putting a substance in the body in a high concentration that doesn't belong there naturally. But the primary reason I bring this up is back to this point about what we consider normal and what we allow to become part of our daily routines. Many of today's generation may not remember, but fifty years ago, smoking was commonplace, almost to the point of being considered normal. Movie stars glamorized smoking on movie screens; doctors endorsed them in magazine ads; and cigarette smoking was allowed in places of work, meeting rooms, hotels, restaurants, high schools, airplanes, bars, parks, and, in some areas of the United States, even hospitals. Pretty much everywhere. Commercials were on TV and in magazines to sell cigarettes, and marketing ran amok per the actual magazine ad below.

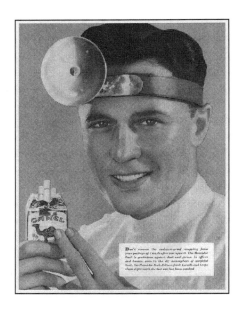

Because of years of public awareness of the health implications, cigarettes are now largely stigmatized and banned from most public areas. This was a long hard battle for consumers to finally win. There were endless studies and counter-studies to prove whether or not smoking was correlated with cancer rates. We look at this now as somewhat absurd. How could putting smoke in your lungs day after day for years *not* affect health? Why was it so hard to come to this conclusion and finally start to push back on corporate marketing related to something that affects our health?

The problem we face as parents is that overconsumption of sugar and the resulting problems are *not* stigmatized. Except for our doctors telling us at the annual examination that our children probably need to *change their diet and get more exercise*, there is very little grassroots effort challenging the status quo on product marketing as it relates to sugar consumption and our children's health. There are families aware and individually making an effort to avoid sugar.

Generally speaking, however, most Americans and people in other developed countries accept it as normal. We are continuing to buy into the marketing frenzy and madness. Are we willing as a society to accept having unhealthy children as OK? At what point do we as consumers challenge this? Maybe it is not acceptable. Maybe this should not be considered normal.

You may be one of those parents who says, "Yes, sometimes I give my little one sweets, but not all of the time, so this doesn't pertain to me." The response again is simple. Your child is likely getting too much sugar all of the time (without added sweets), even though you don't realize it. Manufacturers put sugar in everything, especially for children. Most baby snacks, and even some baby formulas, already contain added sugar. If your children are eating breads, muffins, crackers, snack foods (even foods that don't seem like they would be sweet), and fruits (or drinking fruit juices), they are already getting lots of sugar. If they are snacking on finger food, they are most likely getting sugar. Sweet items you give *sometimes* have more sugar added on top of what they are already getting, making them more dangerous to your children's supply of life money.

Interestingly, veterinarians are also seeing higher rates of type 2 diabetes in pets, which can be attributed to the trends in high-sugar pet snacks. Pet stores have display racks that look like your corner cupcake bakery with loads of sugary snacks for dogs. Kibble for cats is loaded with carbs. Our pets are as vulnerable to this trend as our children!

Let's look at some facts to better understand the extent of this situation and how *abnormal* normal is when it comes to sugar consumption.

How Does Sugar Work?

How does sugar actually work in the body? I'm going to
stay away from the technical jargon and complexity for
those who do not have a medical background. If you are
a doctor or a biologist, yes, you know there is a lot more
to the story. But very simply, sugar is a molecule used to
create energy in cells. It does this in a series of intricate
steps that aren't much different from how cars use gas to
power an engine. When gas and oxygen come together
with a catalyst (a spark), there is combustion, which
creates a reaction called an explosion. This explosion
creates the energy that moves the pistons, which
contributes to the chain of mechanical steps that push
your car forward. The explosion is caused by a
rearrangement of the electrons to form new compounds
in a lower energy state.

In the body, the same sort of reaction happens, but
instead of gas and oxygen, the reaction is with sugar and
oxygen. We consume the sugar in our diet, and the
oxygen we absorb through our lungs. Your cells make
catalysts that initiate these tiny (very tiny!) reactions,
much like a spark. Instead of letting all the electrons
react at once as in an explosion, however, the body
controls the reaction by moving the electrons one at a
time (called the electron transport chain), which creates
controlled energy for the cell to use. The sugar
essentially donates electrons, which are used by cells to
make energy; then oxygen accepts the electrons when
your body is done with them. In your car, the output of

the reaction is water and carbon monoxide. In your body, the output is water and carbon dioxide, which we breathe out.

An analogy for the electron transport chain is how a millpond works. A millpond leverages the force of gravity and the weight of scoops of water one at a time to turn an axle connected to a device that creates energy to grind wheat in a controlled way. Your body uses electron transport chain to power enzymes which then move protons across a barrier where they are then used, one at a time, to power and turn a tiny (very tiny!) turbine, which makes a molecule called ATP that cells use for energy to give us life.

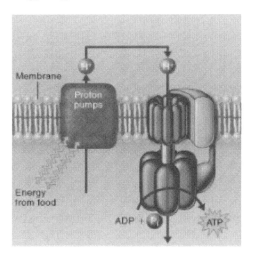

Nature's amazing turbine engine. Quantum Power!

If it weren't for the electron transport chain, all the electrons would react instantly in the cell, creating an explosion. It wouldn't be very healthy to have the trillions of cells that make up the body exploding at once, so our bodies control this automatically by manipulating the use of the electrons.

Sugar is a fuel, just like gasoline. So how much fuel is the right amount? In a car the engine knows how much to use by how much you push the gas pedal. When we go to the pump for gas, we get enough to fill our tank. Now, what would happen if you went to fill your car with gas but didn't stop when the tank was full? You'd just keep pumping more and more gas into the car whether it needed it or not. But the gas is not allowed to overflow onto the pavement and has to stay somewhere in the car. What happens? If your car were able to adjust to its environment, it might come up with a way to convert the gas into something different so that it could store it. In the body, that something is called fat.

It does this in anticipation that the fat will one day be converted to useful energy when necessary. Throughout our evolution, eating a diet high in carbohydrates didn't always come so easily, so this ability to convert sugar to fat—and vice versa—was very handy. But today, most people typically do not create enough energy to burn the calories consumed. This is the start of being overweight and can lead to obesity. Metabolism and genetics also play important parts in how well we burn the calories, and that is a consideration. It is sort of interesting, however, that obesity doesn't exist in countries that do not have unrestricted access to fatty and sugary foods, or whose cultures simply don't embrace them. What we pump in doesn't just magically disappear, even though we like to hope that it does.

When cells use oxygen to create energy there is a side effect called oxidation, which results in unstable molecules inside of the cell. These molecules, called free radicals, have to be neutralized by the immune system or they can be dangerous and cause extensive cellular damage. We'll discuss free radicals and antioxidants later in the book. It is important to note that because of having to manage free radical damage, along with other factors, such as altering the balance between good and bad bacteria in the digestive tract, high sugar consumption puts additional stress on the immune system. This could be having a negative impact on the health of your child.

Another factor is that sugar consumption triggers the pancreas to produce insulin, the hormone that is required to carry the sugar molecule to the cells through the bloodstream. Most hormones can be toxic in unnecessary amounts, making them harmful to cells over time. (Part of why men produce less testosterone later in life when they no longer need it in ample supply, despite what they might think.) If you are overconsuming sugar, the cells can become resistant to the insulin, creating a precursor to type 2 diabetes called insulin resistance. If we are creating substantial amounts of insulin to carry sugar to cells, and the cells do not need that sugar, we are populating the body with unnecessary gasoline, unnecessary hormones, along with resistance to the hormones, which causes an unnecessary chemical mess inside the body. This can happen in our children meal after meal and snack after snack if we are not conscious of what they are consuming.

The important takeaway is that how we interact with our environment plays a significant role in our health, especially for children. Overconsumption of sugary products has become the leading cause of this problem. Why is that?

The Concentration Equation

We discussed earlier what is considered normal. If we look at the lifestyles of our parents and their parents, we could argue that sugary products have been around for a long time and giving them to children is normal and acceptable behavior. Going out for ice cream and having sweet treats for children is almost endemic in America and has been since the first soda pop or bowl of ice cream was served. To point to this as a danger to children on a par with cigarette smoking seems absurd. What has changed?

Food items in high concentration extracted from a solvent (in nature the solvent is usually water) are pretty much a human-made phenomenon. In fact, we have taken it to the extreme where we extract the water from processed food items but then charge three dollars to buy recycled water in bottles! Food items that grow in nature have high water content, which makes them healthier and easier for the body to digest. We sometimes forget that breads, muffins, crackers, bagels, and all bread-related items come from manufacturing plants and do not grow on trees or in gardens.

The *concentration equation* is what I use to describe the dramatic change over the last several decades affecting our children's health as it relates to sugar consumption. Sugar is a molecule that the body craves. It is not much different from an opiate like heroin or a stimulant like cocaine in that when it is consumed, it triggers a positive reaction in a pleasure zone in the brain. Drugs usually work by mimicking a chemical compound that manipulates the brain's response hormones, affecting its activity. Heroin mimics endorphins, which are released in the brain, affecting its pleasure zones. Because heroin massively amplifies dopamine activity, it tricks the brain into feeling an overwhelming pleasure. This immense influx of dopamine causes the brain to function and respond differently, and eventually the user builds a tolerance. The user needs to continue supplementing his or her brain with the drug to feel the same effect and without it goes into intense physical and psychological withdrawal. This is why heroin is so addictive.

Consuming sugar also affects the pleasure zones in the brain (specifically the nucleus accumbens) by releasing dopamine. One study demonstrated that "rats with intermittent access to sugar water will drink in a binge-like manner that releases extracellular dopamine in the nucleus accumbens each time, like the classic effect of most substances of abuse. The consequently leads to changes in the expression or availability of extracellular dopamine receptors." This craving is most likely genetically programmed into our physiology. As I described earlier, sugars and associated molecules are critical to life. In fact, sugar is so elemental to life that genes are even made from it. DNA stands for deoxyribonucleic acid, which is composed of a sugar compound called deoxyribose. Since these molecules weren't always so easy to come by, evolution favored having a positive neurophysiological response in the brain when they were consumed.

Now that researchers understand the science and chemistry of how sugar and other compounds work in the brain, it becomes easy to see how manufacturers manipulate consumers based on this natural craving. If you pump a food product full of sugar, it will sell. S_1 of our three Ss. (You can also pump food full of salt, which the body craves for some of the same reasons. S_2 of our three Ss.)

But, you may point out that sugar exists in most things naturally. It is in fruit, for instance, and all sorts of natural sources. How is that different? This is where the concentration equation comes in.

Two things have been happening simultaneously that affect this equation. One is that manufacturers have continued to figure out ways to concentrate higher and higher amounts of sugar in their products. This is the same concept as turning opium into heroin. In sugar it is done with things like high-fructose corn syrup, zeroing in like a laser beam on the pleasure zone in a child's brain.

For example, a slice of watermelon obviously has sugar in it that makes it taste sweet. This is evolutionary in that when an animal eats the fruit, it disperses the seeds, which is a symbiotic relationship between the plant and animals that consume it. This is the same with all fruits. The difference is that over the course of evolution, the plant doesn't make more sugar than required to encourage an animal to consume the fruit. (The body is efficient; all life is as efficient as possible because creating molecules like sugar takes energy, which in life is precious and is used as sparingly as possible.) Nature is balanced by evolution, access to nutrients, and its environment. To a horse that lives off a diet of hay, a carrot is considered a tasty treat even though not many children would consider a carrot as dessert, unless of course it is carrot cake.

When you consume a slice of watermelon, you are getting mostly water and other healthy molecules—vitamins and antioxidants—along with some carbohydrates like sugar. To quantify, for every one hundred grams of watermelon, you are getting approximately six grams of sugar.

Now let's look at a cupcake, for which there is no need to be efficient since energy production is easier for humans at the top of the food chain. We can concentrate as much sugar as possible in that cupcake to light up those pleasure zones in a child's brain. In contrast to a slice of watermelon, the frosting alone on a cupcake has sixty-three grams of sugar per every one hundred grams. While a slice of watermelon has 6 percent concentration of sugar, the frosting on a cupcake has 63 percent concentration of sugar. A big difference! Never mind the cake part of the cupcake, which is also packed with sugar. Take away the filter of the parent to control the consumption, and it is easy to see why children scarf down these highly concentrated sugary products.

What isn't easy to see is how this is seriously overproducing dopamine in their brains, which leads to side effects just like with a drug. Almost every product today has added sugar, and often it is highly concentrated, which is a key selling tool. The product with the highest concentration of sugar is the one that will most tap the pleasure circuits of the brain. It ends up being the best seller, which encourages competing products to do the same, and we end up with a war between manufacturers to see which one can concentrate the most sugar into its products. It's like an ongoing nuclear arms race, and our children are the victims of the fallout.

Now let's factor in the other part of the equation. Sugar circulates through the bloodstream like other molecules we consume. Obviously the bigger we are, the more mass we have, which means we have a higher volume of blood pumping through our bodies. An average male who weighs 185 pounds has approximately 6,300 mL of blood. When we consume a food product, and it is broken down into its basic components, like the sugar molecule, the concentration in our bloodstream depends on the volume of blood, how long it takes the product to be digested, along with our metabolism (ability to put the sugar to work) and other factors.

Now let's look at this for a child. An average four-year-old weighing forty pounds has approximately 1,400 mL of blood volume. When he or she consumes a food product, there is a significantly higher concentration of the basic components, like the sugar molecule, circulating in the bloodstream. To put it in perspective, imagine taking a gallon of gasoline, pouring it into a bathtub, and then filling up the tub the rest of the way with water. Consider the concentration. Now take a gallon of gasoline, pour it into your bathroom sink, and finish filling it with water. The second scenario would be much more concentrated. Similarly, in the body, different concentration levels have an impact on other factors. In the gasoline example, how much vapor is being given off in the different scenarios that could cause an explosion if exposed to a flame? Would you be willing to drop a match into a bathtub containing of a gallon of gasoline with the rest water? What about your bathroom sink with a gallon of gasoline and the rest water?

If you factor in that higher concentrations of sugar are being added to products, and those products are marketed to younger and younger consumers (which translates into lower blood volumes), it is easy to see how the concentration levels of sugar are becoming higher in our children, affecting their health. In our parents' (or most likely in their parents') day, processed foods were not so readily available, and families generally ate more well-rounded diets with plenty of vegetables. At that time a child might occasionally consume something sugary, for instance, when grandparents took them for ice cream at the state fair. But in today's world, everything children eat has sugar in it. Most children are already eating way too many carbohydrates just in their regular meals, never mind added sweets. Furthermore, children start eating sugary products at much younger ages, largely because of corporate marketing.

Without considering the consequences of this equation, consumers around the world are being manipulated and are accepting it as normal. In the United States, it is embarrassing how blatantly soft drink and candy companies advertise to children at places like movie theaters or on children's television shows. If you take your children to see the newest animated movie (which I love just as much as my kids do, by the way), you can expect to sit through several soft-drink commercials telling you to please be quiet, turn off your cell phone, and gulp their products from barrel-size cups.

It isn't just in the United States. I remember being in Lima, Peru, at a large shopping mall during Christmas. In the center they set up a stage with a show with Christmas music and elves and reindeer and an option for children to visit Santa Claus. Hundreds of families were seated all around the stage. Turns out the show was sponsored by a soft-drink company, and the children had the chance to come on stage and meet Santa and get a free can of soft drink, which earned them a jolly "Ho! Ho! Ho!" and celebration and applause. The theme was "The Taste of Christmas." This is blatant marketing manipulation aimed at children that we allow to creep too easily into our families' lives. Below is an older magazine advertisement with Santa helping sell cigarettes. Sound familiar?

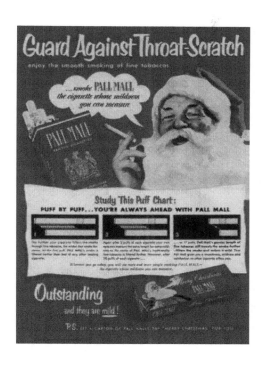

The Portion/Proportion Problem

So how does the concentration equation affect us? Part of it comes down to another challenge I call the portion/proportion problem. Usually, serving sizes are based on consumption by adults. A twelve-ounce can of soda, for instance, has approximately thirty-nine grams of sugar per can. For an adult male, the American Heart Association recommends no more than thirty-eight grams of sugar *per day*. An adult has already gone over the maximum recommendation with just one can of a soft drink. Never mind taking into consideration that most do not consume soft drinks in twelve-ounce sizes anymore. It is not surprising to see drink containers twice this size!

What is the impact on a child who has a much smaller mass and blood volume? Basic physics and our equation above tell us that if a child is half the mass of an adult, the saturation level in the bloodstream will be double for the same amount of a given substance. This affects not only the amount of sugar, caffeine, fats, and other unhealthy ingredients, but it also has chemical implications, such as a change in blood pH levels. When we give them adult-size portions of ice cream, muffins, soda, or other sugary products, we are essentially giving them double or quadruple of what we are getting for the same portion. This is a major flaw in how we measure consumption.

One of the first considerations in a health strategy for children is to rethink how we handle portions of food items, especially those that are unhealthy. Food manufacturers rarely make portions appropriate for children. In fact, the opposite has happened. Now most candy bars come in "sharing sizes," which means they are essentially double the serving size (and are very rarely shared). In many places, children even have the option of "all you can consume" like we see at some yogurt franchises or with fountain-drink stands in restaurants.

Without putting filters in place, who controls the level of consumption? Parents may try, but it's usually too late. Have you ever caught yourself saying to your child, "You've had two cookies already, and that is enough." Actually half a cookie was probably enough because that cookie was sized for an adult and not for a child. The younger the child, the fewer adult sugary products he or she should be consuming. But we usually don't think about it this way. Rethinking the impact that portions have on our children and how we are managing this as parents is a great first step.

Impact on Self-Esteem

All loving parents want their children to be healthy and happy. No parent wants to see his or her children being bullied or picked on for being different. Being overweight is one of those factors that leads kids to being bullied, which can have devastating consequences on their self-esteem. Schools and communities go to great lengths to put programs in place to offset the consequences of bullying and create an environment that is safe and inclusive for all children. There is no question that some children have slower metabolisms and other physiological conditions that will dispose them to being overweight. It is sad and frustrating to see children getting picked on for conditions they cannot control.

However, there are children with weight problems that could be controlled by the parents. I see lots of parents dropping off their children at school or walking around the grocery store wearing workout clothes, looking like they are heading to or just coming from the gym. Parents tend to go through cycles of trying to get into better health habits, but are they promoting the same standards in their children? Are their children overweight and this is being accepted as OK by the parents? Are we being consistent in the health expectations we set as a family? These are important questions that parents can ask themselves just to understand their baseline.

The Sugar Traps

The "Sugar-Free" Facade

When it comes to sugar traps, one marketing term we need to be careful of is *sugar-free*. First, there doesn't need to be such a thing as sugar-free, because as we discussed earlier in the book, the body needs sugar to make energy. The sugar intake just needs to be in the right amounts. The problem comes from overconsumption, which is a different issue to solve. What the sugar-free marketing is trying to do is satisfy your child's sugar craving by developing manufactured versions of sugar that appeal to taste buds and brain chemistry but have less impact on the body. Most artificial sweeteners work because your body doesn't recognize the modified molecules, which cannot be digested, so they are eliminated as waste.

This may work in theory but not in practice. Sugary products are usually unhealthy for many different reasons, so children still ingest things they shouldn't be eating, even if they are getting less sugar. It is also difficult to know the health implications of these modified sugar-like molecules. This is just looking for a different way to feed the same bad craving without making the changes necessary to address the root of the problem. Artificial sweeteners are the methadone of sugary products. It helps ease parents' consciences to think they are being more responsible by giving these products to their children. But if our children are addicted to sweet products, they will go right back to

bad eating habits when they have the option to make their own purchasing decisions. The best way to get your children to eat less sugar is to break the sugar habit, not try to find a work-around.

The Kids' Menu

In my other book, I have a section about kids' menus and how unhealthful they tend to be, and the same applies to feeding the sugar addiction. Unfortunately, the children's menu at most restaurants offers food that is almost never healthful. Children's items that are common for even the most respectable franchise restaurants include

- spaghetti or other pasta;
- chicken fingers with fries;
- pizza;
- hot dog; and
- cheeseburger with fries.

Almost all carbs. Along with this you'll find complimentary dessert items with kids' menus, and most meals include unlimited amounts of soft drink. As parents, we have to be conscious of what our children are ordering at restaurants and ensure we are being consistent. The best strategy is to skip the kids' menu and order something healthful for children from the adult menu, which will often have much better options.

Pacifier Turns to Agitator

It is easy for parents to fall into the habit of using sugary food as a pacifier for young children. As a parent, I understand the temptation to give children something to snack on that keeps them happy (and quiet). Sometimes they come back for seconds and are able to get additional sugary items. Other times they are not permitted second helpings, which may cause children to get upset and throw a tantrum. Children may throw tantrums at the grocery store when they want an unhealthy product, but the parent resists. What is the best way to address this problem?

The first and most obvious way is to prevent them from being exposed to sugary products in the first place, especially at an early age. Why do we even open our homes and let these products in? The longer a child can go without being exposed, the better. This may sound unreasonable to many parents because, as I've pointed out, sugary products are so ingrained in our culture that we accept giving them to children as normal, especially items like cookies, cupcakes, crackers, chips, cereals, yogurts, ice cream, hard candy, and candy bars.

As parents, we can first ask ourselves what nutritional value these items provide to help keep our children healthy. What impact does the product have on their bodies and brain chemistries? How does the *input* affect the *output*? The items I list above usually offer no nutritional value beyond carbs, which children tend to get plenty of without snacks. As I have mentioned, the sugar also affects brain chemistry just like a drug. The next question should be, "Why would I give it to them?" It is an important question that parents must ask themselves.

Once a child is exposed to sugar, or any other chemical compound that affects his or her neural chemistry, the brain literally changes, perhaps permanently. Our wonderfully efficient brains are quick to learn, for better or worse, based on behavior and environmental stimuli. The brain has memorized that something sugary is going to release dopamine and affect its pleasure zones.

Because of this, the best approach is to try not to expose children to highly concentrated sugary products for as long as possible. Fruits and vegetables are different because the sugars are natural so they are not as highly concentrated, and they offer other nutritional value that is beneficial to the body. But the higher concentrations have a more profound impact.

These decisions are typically made at the grocery store, because if it isn't in your pantry, then the child cannot eat it. It is best to try to ban these snack items. Again, I know this sounds extreme to many parents, but it has gotten to the point where these types of filters are necessary to protect our children's health. Not exposing them to these products has a few advantages for the parent:

1. The longer you can keep them from being exposed, the longer you have to instill better eating habits. Given the choice between eating vegetables or throwing a small fit to get a highly concentrated sugary alternative, what does a child most likely choose? It is easy for parents to go down the path of least resistance and fold to a crying child who is trying to get ahold of something sugary. This creates a precedent that can be difficult to break. Who is training whom?
2. Additional time gives their internal organs and systems, such as the endocrine and immune systems, time to develop before being exposed to a lot of sugar. As we pointed out, environmental influences and early exposure to different food items play roles in how these systems develop and how we are affected by psychological cravings.
3. Studies have shown that early childhood exposure to sugar can have a permanent effect on eating habits. This is linked to how certain molecules, such as glucose, affect our brains and body chemistries, and how we respond to those changes.

But let's say that we put these filters within our home. A problem for many parents is the sugary food at birthday parties or other events. One way to solve this is to bring your own food items that are healthier for a smaller child. I see many parents do this for children who need gluten- or dairy-free food. I know this is hard for parents and their children when most of the kids get the sugary stuff, and they give their child something different to eat.

***

As a child grows older, you could consider using the "by-half" rule. Cut sugary items by half or even a third. This pertains to things like muffins or cookies or other products bought at the grocery store or on-the-go restaurants or chains. The question then becomes what to do with the leftovers. Of course, you can eat whatever is left—which I do myself sometimes, even though I know it isn't healthy for me, either! The best thing, however, is to throw it away. This may seem like a waste of money and food, but in this situation, the irony is that wasting the money is actually a better investment.

Let me put it like this. If you pay fifty dollars for gasoline but can only put twenty-five dollars in your tank, what is the safest way to manage the excess? Do you continue to pump the gasoline all over the ground at the pumping station? Doesn't this create a more dangerous situation than just stopping at twenty-five dollars and accepting the financial loss? Being the consumer gives us the flexibility to dictate the serving size, which isn't always related to cost or value.

Sugar Disguised as Healthy

Another trap that is easy to fall into is giving sugar to our children in foods that we think are healthful. There are many products that advertise health benefits in the big print, but when you actually read the ingredients, you find they are full of sugar and other processed ingredients. Below are some that parents need to be careful with.

Juices (such as orange juice)—Parents are taught to think that fruit juice is healthful, which is misleading. Most of the real nutrition, such as fiber or antioxidants, have been removed from commercial juices during processing. Pasteurization damages antioxidants and other beneficial compounds. Almost all that is left is highly concentrated sugar water. For example, to get the same amount of orange juice as in one glass, a child would need to eat approximately ten oranges. This is obviously much more than they would consume if they were actually eating the fruit.

If you are in the habit of giving fruit juice to your children, one strategy to help manage the sugar is to dilute the juice with water. This doesn't have to be done all at once and can be adjusted a little bit at a time so your child doesn't notice and complain.

Bread—Bread is another food item parents have been taught is healthful, which is also misleading. Most bread today is loaded with sugar. In fact, it is difficult to find a bread option that does not have sugar added. Some sugar may be necessary to give the bread flavor, but consumers need to be careful to read the ingredients and look for bread that has low sugar. When children get used to sugary bread, it can be difficult to move them to healthier options, so it is best to get accustomed to lower-sugar options from the start. Another option for DIY'ers is to bake your bread in the home, which helps control the ingredients.

Yogurt—Most commercial yogurts are basically just desserts. You can ignore the health benefits advertised, such as it being a probiotic. I discussed probiotics at length in my other book and won't go into detail here, but this term is essentially just a marketing phrase without a lot of science to back up the health benefits. We have been getting probiotics from our diet for millions of years without having to manipulate it in our foods. If your children are eating a healthy diet, they are getting the probiotics and prebiotics they need daily.

If you want your child to get the health benefits of yogurt, then the best strategy is to buy pure, unsweetened yogurt and add ingredients such as honey or fruit to give it more flavor. You can mash blueberries, for instance, which makes for a healthier alternative to commercial prepackaged yogurts. Be careful not to fall into the trap of thinking that Greek yogurt is healthier than regular yogurt. Along with all the sugar, most commercial Greek yogurts add modified cornstarch and other ingredients that compromise the health benefits.

Sports drinks—The overconsumption of sports drinks by young children (who may or may not play sports) has turned into a leading sugar enabler in today's suburban world. Despite all the jargon about electrolytes and other health benefits, these drinks are essentially just sugar water. You may be led to believe that children need these carbs after exercise. OK. But most children get plenty of carbs from all the other stuff they eat. All they usually need after exercise is hydration. By developing the habit of drinking sports drinks, they are getting more and more hooked on sugary drinks, and it becomes more ingrained. Not only are you having to stop them from drinking soft drinks at home, but also now they are drinking sports drinks after a little bit of physical activity. Because sports drinks feed the craving and are associated with something that is typically considered healthful (sports), they easily slip into the daily routine and consumption pattern and continue to feed the sugar addiction.

This doesn't mean that a child should never drink a sports drink or that sports drinks do not help in certain situations related to exercise. Sports-drink consumption has to be taken in context with some common sense applied. Here in Florida, where we live, for instance, Donovan Darius, former wide receiver from the Jacksonville Jaguars, runs a camp every year for young football players learning the sport. The camp lasts three afternoons for several hours and is an intense workout, amplified by the late-summer Florida sun. In this situation, drinking a sports drink probably makes sense in order to get carbs and electrolytes back into the body.

But young children, playing forty minutes of organized flag football or soccer on Saturday morning, probably don't need to drink a bottle of a sports drink. It is just about awareness. As parents, we must learn to be more conscious of where sugar (and especially disguised sugar) is creeping into our daily routines so we can manage it appropriately.

Granola anything—Almost all granola products are laced with sugar, sugar by-products, or other ingredients that have sugar, such as chocolate or yogurt pieces. If a child actually ate only a piece of granola, he or she would spit it out. Granola bars and products are just concentrated sugar snacks that need to be managed carefully.

Cereals—Children's cereal is usually full of sugar, in addition to the sugar in the milk. There are a lot of healthier options available, but it is important to read the label and make sure you are buying cereal that is low in sugar. Consumers have to be careful with the advertising, as cereal companies often will advertise added ingredients as being healthy even though they are not. Some examples are clusters or flakes of granola, yogurt, or dried fruit. These added items are usually just processed little packages of added sugar. Manufacturers are always trying to stay one step ahead of consumers and will hide the fact that their products are full of sugar in different ways. Another trick is touting honey in the advertising. This usually means a flavoring to make it taste like honey, combined with lots of sugar. They also do the same with cinnamon.

As an example, regular Cheerios has one gram of sugar per serving. A serving of its cousin counterpart, Honey Nut Cheerios, on the other hand, has nine grams of sugar. There is little to no health benefit from the honey aspect of this because of the processing, but your child is getting nine times the amount of sugar per serving! They also do the same things with the ancient-grains version of the cereal, which has five grams of sugar per serving. Using ancient grains as a marketing hook sounds great, but a different grain doesn't mean the product is any healthier, especially if the sugar has to go up by five times. But sweet sells. It is just another way to sell a more sugary version while sounding healthier to parents.

One way to get around this is to reinvent how you serve cereal in your home. You can make a healthier bowl of cereal by buying cereal that is low in sugar and then adding your own ingredients. For instance, if you want to make it a little sweeter, you can add real honey. Pure honey is a natural antioxidant and has a lot of health properties. You can also add your own cinnamon and/or fresh-cut fruit, like strawberries or blueberries. This way you can balance how much is going into the cereal and the sugar concentration levels.

If your child is in the habit of making their own cereal in the mornings, you can have fruit already cut in the right portions available in the refrigerator that they can add. The child will not usually cut their own fresh fruit to add to the cereal. This is an opportunity to help them get additional vitamins while supplementing their cereal with something fresh and healthy, instead of getting it from an additive in the product.

Don't forget that milk is also full of sugar (and fat), so be careful with that as well. One option is to substitute unsweetened almond milk for cow's milk. Your little one might notice this, so you may choose to do it a little at a time. You could use half cow's milk and half almond milk to start with, for instance, or find a proportion that works in the short term while weaning him or her off cow's milk.

There are also sugary products that are healthful, but we have to be careful with them. Below are some examples.

Bananas—The bananas in grocery stores today are so genetically modified that they are almost twice the size of the typical bananas that used to grow on trees in the wild. Because of this, along with being in captivity on a regimented diet, the monkeys in zoos were becoming type 2 diabetics from eating them on a regular basis. (Sorry, the biologist in me is coming out.) Zoo officials had to change the diet of monkeys in captivity, so they now eat primarily greens and other healthful items, and no more bananas.

What does that say about bananas and our children? Bananas have a lot of sugar, and the larger the bananas, the more the sugar concentration. One positive with bananas is that the sugar takes a while to digest and get into the bloodstream, so the sugar impact is more spread out over the course of the banana's digestion, unlike the sugar in dates or raisins, which hits the bloodstream fast and in higher concentration. However, we still need to be careful not to think that bananas are a healthful way to feed a child's craving for sugar. Better than a candy bar but still high in sugar. Maybe this is where the by-half rule is applicable. Maybe we can start giving half a banana or several small slices in a small bowl instead of the whole banana.

Low-fat items—Typically, when we see the words "low fat" on food products, it's just synonymous with "high sugar." The main point is that fat and sugar are reciprocal, meaning that sugar turns into fat as a means of storage if the sugar is not burned through activity. When we consume low-fat items, all we are essentially doing is substituting one thing for another and falsely assuming it is better. From a health perspective, low-fat products are just as unhealthy as their higher-fat counterparts unless the child is active enough to burn the calories consumed from the added sugar.

Gluten-free—Every few years a new marketing term comes out to help sell food products. For the last few years, this has been the gluten-free craze. Granted there are clinical studies demonstrating the physical and mental impacts on children from the overconsumption of gluten products. I'm not suggesting that some children are not allergic to gluten or that putting them on a gluten-free diet doesn't benefit them. The only point is that manufacturers are using the gluten-free craze to sell products by just loading them with more sugar. Replacing gluten-free food with high-sugar alternatives may not be the best answer for the long-term health of the child.

Cutting Sugar from Your Children's Diet

Put Filters in Place

Filters are a constant part of life, even though we sometimes forget about them. They are in the air-conditioning units in our houses, our cars, Internet access, water systems, and so on. All these systems we use daily have filters in place to help protect us and our families from elements that could harm us. Yet it is interesting that we usually do not put filters on our pantries and refrigerators. Children have unlimited access to products like soft drinks, cookies, crackers, chips, and other concentrated items, which can lead to bad eating habits that are hard to break.

Very often I hear parents say, "I wish my children liked healthier foods, but they won't eat them," which I always find puzzling. We don't let our children do other dangerous things just because they want to or to avoid having them throw a fit, so why should unhealthful eating habits be any different? The smart approach is for our children to consume what parents decide is good for them, not what they think tastes good. If you have unhealthful snack items within grabbing reach, then most likely your children are helping themselves.

If you consider it in more detail, your pantry is the end of a long supply chain aimed at your children—from processing plants in Latin America, where sugar is extracted from sugarcane and bleached, and the chemical elements are manipulated into more concentrated variants, to the manufacturing plants in China, where the syrups are combined with lots of other unhealthy ingredients and packaged with child-friendly branding and stamped with today's best-known action hero. Then these snacks are shipped around the planet and stored in distribution centers to be delivered to store shelves. Because of the advertisements embedded in their favorite children's shows or games they play on mobile devices, they end up in your pantry. All along this supply chain, is there ever one stop gate that says, "Hmm, maybe children shouldn't be eating this because it is not healthful?" Unfortunately, there is not. The only filter, the only voice of reason, the only one concerned about the long-term health of your child is you, the parent or guardian. You are often the last and only reliable filter.

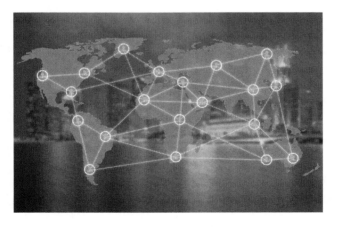

Looking at your pantry from the company's perspective

You can tell a lot about the health habits of your family just by doing an inventory of the pantry: half-eaten bags of chips and cookies, easily available to children of all ages, and half-consumed two-liter bottles of soft drinks, also easily available to children of all ages. These are signs of a home without sugar filters.

One of the first and most effective steps toward breaking the sugar habit for your children is to ensure you are putting the right filters in place. Imagine, for instance, that on your pantry and refrigerator there were larger filters that only let out things that were good for you and your family. This is especially important for sugary products and snack items. Look at what you have in your pantry or refrigerator currently. What would get filtered, and what would get through? This applies to what they eat *and* drink. It applies to the pantry *and* the refrigerator. You can significantly reduce your child's sugar consumption just by being an effective filter within your home.

Be Careful with Concentrated Food Items

We are not always available to monitor what our children eat. One way to address this is to ensure we are controlling what is available for them when we are not watching. As I mentioned previously, concentrated food items for children are a leading cause of the bad eating habits affecting their health. If we stock fewer concentrated products and more fruits and vegetables, they will not have those options available. The best way to keep your child out of the cookie jar is to get rid of the cookie jar. This sounds like common sense, but many parents struggle with this. How do you prevent having unhealthy foods in your pantry, and what are the right foods that should be available for children to consume?

The Pen Is Stronger than the Pantry

The best way to address this is to go back to working from a defined grocery list that focuses on health, instead of making impromptu purchases at the grocery store. Many parents use lists, but usually for those basic items such as eggs and milk. One would hardly see a box of individually packaged Oreo cookies, a dozen donuts, and three two-liter bottles of soda pop on a grocery list, although nowadays I think soft drinks are so commonly accepted they probably do make it on a lot of lists. Still, those are items we tend to toss into our grocery carts and store in our pantries without a lot of thought. The best way to change purchasing behavior is with accountability. Write your list before you go to the store, which will cause additional scrutiny and help you manage purchasing decisions. When possible, do not take your children grocery shopping with you. Taking them shopping only advocates purchases based on what they are craving, which can be manipulated through product placement on aisles and shelves. Companies intentionally spend a premium for those shelf spaces so they are seen by children. Notice where the high-sugar cereals are in this photo from an example grocery-store aisle?

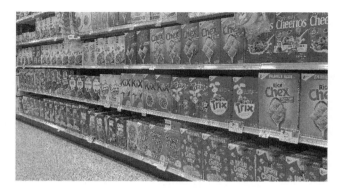

Another thing parents can do to be empowered and make better decisions is to keep a journal of their children's intake over a short time. For one week, write down a brief list of what they consume. Then you have something you can work with. This doesn't have to be a complex exercise. It can be as simple as keeping a notebook in your kitchen and writing down what and when. Most people are surprised when they make the effort and see all the foods their children have eaten that they tend to forget about or don't consider, especially related to sweets. Eating is one of the most habit-based activities of our lives, and habits are easy to overlook, causing us not to scrutinize the underlying behavior, which is part of what makes them a habit in the first place. Once you have this journal, you can do an analysis.

For example, let's say you review this journal and find your child likes to snack on a particular food item every day when he or she gets home from school. What exactly is in this snack item? Have you read the ingredients carefully? Does it list sugar in some form as a primary ingredient? The ingredients for products are listed by most of the first ingredient listed first, and then the next ingredient, and so on. Very often sugar, or a variant, is the first or second ingredient. Is there a way you could switch their favorite after-school snack with something a little healthier?

This change in behavior doesn't have to be effected overnight. Another mistake parents make is to try to force children into better eating habits too quickly when they are already accustomed to bad eating habits. Forcing a change too soon tends to be met with resistance, which is often a frustrating battle for the parents. It is usually more effective to change gradually, according to a strategy. Let's discuss ideas for this approach.

Healthier Snack Alternatives

I understand replacing sugary snacks with healthier alternatives isn't easy. Four-year-olds accustomed to sugary snacks have acquired a taste for them, and like recovering addicts, it is hard for them to satisfy the pleasure zone in their brains when they try to go back to normal food items. Again, don't try to make the change overnight. It is usually more sustainable to make small incremental changes over time. Let's take an example.

Making a better peanut butter and jelly sandwich

Say we review the journal discussed and find our children come home from school every day and want us to make them a peanut butter and jelly sandwich. Not a bad snack if it is made with healthful ingredients. By this, I mean that each one of the three components of a peanut butter and jelly sandwich—bread, jelly, and peanut butter—has a lot of variability in how much sugar is in the sandwich depending on the quality of the components. Most commercial peanut butter brands add sugar to their products. Jellies have a lot of added sugar, along with bread.

What can you do to take a standard after-school snack option and make it healthier over time? Your first option might be to switch your peanut-butter brand to one that does not include added sugar. Chances are your child won't even notice. A lot of grocery stores even allow you to grind your own peanuts or buy freshly ground peanut butter, which doesn't have added ingredients. A popular peanut-butter brand with added sugar, for instance, has three grams of sugar per serving. A comparable brand without added sugar has one gram of sugar per serving. This switch alone reduces the sugar intake from the peanut butter by two-thirds. A good start. Small wins lead to larger victories.

The next option would be to find a jelly without added sugar (but not labeled sugar-free). It is a little ridiculous how much sugar—usually in the form of high-fructose corn syrup or some other highly concentrated sugar—is added to commercial jellies despite the fact that fruit itself is sweet. It is possible to find jellies that do not have added sugar or are sweetened by something more natural, like apple juice. One popular strawberry jelly brand has twelve grams of sugar per serving, and most of this sugar is in the form of high-fructose corn syrup, corn syrup, and sugar. Another that uses apple juice to sweeten it has eleven grams of sugar. Not a big reduction but at least a more natural form of sugar, for what it's worth. This small change reduced the sugar by another gram per serving. Another small win.

The next option would be to reconsider the bread. Unfortunately, bread and bread-related products are one of the biggest areas of concern for added sugar. If you read the ingredients, you'll find sugar is usually listed as the second ingredient behind wheat, which means that it has the second-highest level of concentration in the product. Switching breads can be more difficult because children get used to sugary bread and tend to notice if switched to a healthier option. This might need to be a gradual change. Going from honey wheat to wheat in the same brand, for instance, may reduce sugar without a significant change to texture or taste. One popular brand has two grams of sugar for honey wheat, while the same brand has one gram of sugar for wheat.

But big deal, this is only a one-gram reduction, right? Actually, we have cut the sugar from bread *in half,* which is a big deal. We tend to not apply the same significance to small numbers as we do to large numbers, but the relationship is the same. What if someone told you they could reduce your credit-card debt from $20,000 to $10,000 instantly?

Our original peanut butter and jelly sandwich had seventeen grams of sugar (not counting other carbs), and our slightly adjusted sandwich has thirteen grams of sugar (not counting other carbs). This is about a 27 percent reduction in sugar in just one sandwich without doing anything different besides reconsidering the ingredients.

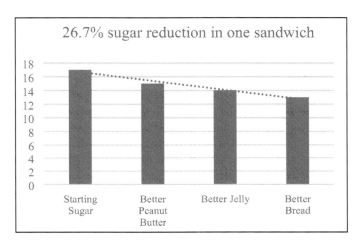

26.7% sugar reduction in one sandwich

Starting Sugar	Better Peanut Butter
Better Jelly	Better Bread

You are probably thinking this is too much fuss just for a peanut butter and jelly sandwich. But it matters over time. One dollar a day doesn't seem like much, but over ten years, it is almost $4,000. In the context of healthful living, small things make a difference and add up. Of course, you can do big things as well, like run a marathon, but if you are getting the smaller things right on a daily basis, that can be just as sustainable for you and your children.

Some other healthful snack ideas

Sliced apples with peanut butter—Red Delicious apples have one of the highest concentrations of antioxidants (as long as they are not peeled), so sliced apple with peanut butter (without added sugar) makes for a pretty good and filling afternoon snack. Another good option is to use almond butter instead of peanut butter. The only thing to watch for in almond butter is added sugar and palm oil. You may have to search a little harder to find pure almond butter that doesn't have added ingredients.

Sliced cucumbers—A lot of children seem to like cucumber that is sliced the long way. Cucumbers are healthful and low in sugar, with a lot of water for hydration. Carrots, red pepper, or any other vegetables, also make for great snack options if they are sliced or cut in a way that makes it easy for the child to eat them. Red pepper has more vitamin C then an orange!

Hummus or other dip with celery, sliced cucumber, sliced carrots, or red peppers—Getting a child to eat a carrot slice can sometimes be a challenge, but a hummus dip can help. Just make sure the hummus is itself healthy and does not have added sugar or other unhealthy ingredients.

Raw nuts – Raw nuts have a lot of healthy properties *as long as they are not roasted and salted.* Pecans, for instance, are loaded with antioxidants. Cashews have zinc which help support the immune system. Almonds have alpha-tacapherol which, based on research, seems to help with heart health.

A great snack choice for children is to buy a variety of raw nuts at the grocery store and then mix them together in a container. This way when the child wants a snack you can put a handful in a small bowl for them. You might also put a few raisins into your nut mix.

Making your own desserts

One way to let your children enjoy sweets while limiting the compromise on health is to make your own dessert items from scratch. This turns out to be easier than it sounds. In fact, it is amazing how healthful you can make desserts if you make them yourself.

To this point it also helps you to see how unhealthful dessert items are that you buy in a store. Take, for instance, an apple pie. If you look up an online recipe for apple pie, it probably has added corn syrup as an ingredient, along with sugar. Corn syrup and sugar together is a lot of sugar to put in your and your children's bodies, even if it is just one piece at a time. I find, however, that I can make an apple pie at home with very little (if any) added sugar. You can add more apples and use almond flour with applesauce (no sugar added) to get a nice consistency for the pie.

I have some recipes on my website at www.jayfoard.com, but they aren't really necessary. Basically the best strategy is to look up different recipes and then work out how to make a healthier alternative. For instance, if the recipe calls for a cup of sugar, try using half a cup or less. One can usually make up for one unhealthful ingredient by using more of something healthy. In apple pie, for instance, you would put less bleached, concentrated sugar but more apple. In cherry pie, more cherries.

Granted, the pie is not going to taste the same as the one

61

you buy at the store, full of corn syrup and preservatives and high amounts of sugar, but it depends on what you let your family become accustomed to.

Since I reference it above, let's take an apple-pie recipe as an example. Below are the ingredients based on a recipe I found online, assuming a store-bought crust.

6–8 medium Granny Smith apples, peeled and sliced
2 tablespoons cornstarch
2 teaspoons cinnamon
1/2 teaspoon salt
2/3 cup sugar
2/3 cup melted butter
2/3 cup light corn syrup
1 teaspoon vanilla
1 tablespoon lemon juice

I played around with the ingredients, modified the recipe, and it now looks like this:

Enough apple slices to fill the pie crust (without peeling the slices—the peel is the most healthful part of the apple)
2 teaspoons cinnamon
1/2 teaspoon salt
Applesauce without added sugar
1/4 cup unsalted butter, melted
1/2 cup almond flour
1/4 cup of light brown sugar
1 teaspoon vanilla

For this recipe I've cut out corn syrup and reduced the amount of sugar from 2/3 cup to 1/4 cup without a big impact on the taste. This recipe is just an example and not to be taken too specifically as I am not a professional cook or chef. My point is that you don't have to follow recipes exactly as they are written if they are compromising the health of your family. To me, using as much sugar or corn syrup in a pie as recommended in online recipes is unnecessary and irresponsible. Unfortunately, we tend to buy goods blindly and follow recipes as written without considering the consequences. But as parents, we have the opportunity to reevaluate what is right for our families and health strategies.

As I pointed out in my last book, people want the silver bullet for better health, but there isn't one. It comes from lifestyle changes, compromises, and finding balance. It comes from doing the small things, like rewriting an apple-pie recipe, and doing the big things, like not putting unhealthful sugary products in our grocery carts while at the store. It comes from constant awareness and being willing to stand up to persuasive marketing by applying basic common sense in purchasing decisions.

Some of it just comes down to relearning what we accept as normal.

Unite with Other Parents

For those who accept the sugar problem and the impact it has on their children's health, it becomes a constant battle trying to prevent overexposure to sugary products. Elementary-school events are a good example. An end-of-year sweet snack for the children based on a year of hard work is more than fair. Instead, what tends to happen is children are inundated with ridiculous amounts of sugary products for pretty much every event all year. And not just a little bit. Cookies, more cookies, more cookies, cupcakes, more cupcakes, chocolates, ice cream in multiple flavors, cake, and more cake. For those who are trying to be conscious of sugar intake for their children, it becomes almost impossible to control. Parents don't want to follow around behind their children taking everything out of their hands before they put it into their mouths.

In my opinion, the first thing needed is an admission that sugar consumption is a major consideration in relation to our children's health and has to be managed by parents. We cannot expect government restrictions to aid in our parenting. They tried this with soft drinks in New York City, to no avail. We also cannot expect corporations to back off their blatant marketing of sugary products to children. In fact, they are only getting more blatant. There needs to be a bottom-up grassroots effort by parents working together to control the madness for the sake of our children's future health. It is one of those "you can't solve a problem if you can't admit there is a problem" problems, and once we admit there is a problem, only we as parents can solve it, working together.

Once we can acknowledge the problem, the best solution is for parents to unite, coordinate, and work together. This way, sweets can be minimized and controlled. If one parent is bringing cupcakes, then other parents do not need to bring cakes, cookies, candy bars, and other unhealthful snacks. The same is important for any function, whether it is a birthday party or an after-school event. The basic fact here is children *do not need all this sugar.* Why do we even make this compromise? When children come together, they are typically enjoying the social aspects of the event anyway. Tables loaded with sugary products are unnecessary in the larger picture. If we work together, we can find better ways to reward our children by just letting them be healthy and social.

Again, this isn't to say that giving a child something sweet every once in a while is a bad thing. Most things are OK in moderation. Our bodies are efficient at using what we put into them and discarding what they do not need. An occasional sweet item, such as a dessert for older children, a treat of frozen yogurt, or a cupcake at a birthday party, will not permanently compromise their health. But if these one-off events become part of their normal routine, then the consequences can be devastating later in life.

Learning to Offset Snacking Behavior

Children are as prone to habits as adults and often snack out of boredom and habit. When we allow our children to snack, what they snack on should not be random. Children quickly learn how to take advantage of this. Random snacking typically means sugary (or salty) snacking, which can become a habit without the parent realizing it. Snacking should be strategic and well thought out so that it aligns with regular meals and schedules.

A place to be conscious that usually encourages bad snacking behavior is in the car. Usually parents will grab or purchase whatever packaged good is available to give a child as they head off to school, practice or other activities. Smart car snacking is a great way to encourage better snacking. You may want to consider this ahead of time so you can plan. If you have cucumber slices or other healthier options already cut then you can grab them easily. If your child won't eat these healthier items then you may consider to just ban snacking in the car, period. From a health perspective, no snacking is a lot better option then bad snacking out of habit or convenience.

One way to control snacking is leveraging the strategy we discussed before about working from a grocery list. If you don't want your child to snack on it, then don't make it available in your pantry. This also helps you control what you are tempted to give your children. If healthful snack items are all that are available, it isn't your fault, and there is nothing you can do about it at that point! If they want a snack, the only option is a healthful alternative or avoid snacking between meals.

ABCs and 123s to Break the Sugar Habit

To make this as simple as possible, I have outlined the ABCs and 123s of breaking the sugar habit. This is a summary to highlight the most important takeaways I've tried to capture in the book.

ABC

A—Always Read the Ingredients

Many parents buy products based on the big print on the front of the box and not based on the small print on the side of the box. Marketing muddles the health topic, making it hard for parents to know what is healthy and what is not. The best way to get around this is to always rely on the small-print ingredients list only. This is where companies are required to put exactly what is in the product you are buying. Try to get into the habit of reading the small-print ingredients on everything you buy until you are familiar with certain ingredients in certain brands and know what is actually in the product. By doing this, you will be able to avoid falling for the big-print advertising and have a much better sense of what you are providing to your children.

B—Be Conscious and Consistent

A lot of managing sugar intake and overall health for our children is just being conscious of what they are eating and what we are feeding them. Learn to think of sugar as a bad thing, not a good thing! Once you come to this realization, then you can start to rethink how and why you let sugar into your children's lives. It is best for this to start when they are young, while we can still control what they are consuming.

If they are older, it may be more difficult to change their eating habits, but it is not too late and still just as important. Parents have to help their children break their sugar habit, and how to do this varies, depending on each family. Whatever strategy parents decide to use, by being conscious and consistent, it makes it easier to sustain a health strategy and keep your children from trying to manipulate you based on sugar cravings.

One way to be consistent is to *set goals* for your children (and perhaps your whole family). If you feel that your child is overweight (or if your pediatrician points it out), you can address this by setting a weight for the child that aligns with your family's goals and the child's health. You can execute against this by having a strategic meal plan that everyone in the home adheres to. Helping our children eat better and healthier usually means the whole family can benefit. The point is don't just accept your child being overweight as a lost cause. With a little bit of work and some goal setting, most parents can take matters into their hands to address the problem.

C—Control Snacking and Eating Habits

Most parents in some way do try to control their
children's diet at mealtime. It tends to be the in-between
times when children spontaneously eat a lot of sugary
products. Examples are random trips for soda and snacks
throughout the day or night. Children snack out of
boredom or nervousness, just as we do. And those
snacks are usually not healthful. Cutting out unhealthy
snacking or replacing those snacks with healthful
options can help streamline sugar intake and make sure
that you are aware of what your children are eating and
how it is affecting their health.

For trips to the *all you can eat* frozen yogurt, soft drink
or other dessert establishments, learn to let a little be
enough, especially for young children. If a child has the
option to determine their own serving size, which is
usually already in an oversized container, they will pile
on the yogurt and toppings until they are running over
the side. As we mentioned, yogurt is full of sugar and
should be considered a dessert item, not a health item. A
parent can easily cut the amount a child puts in their
container by two-thirds and still have a good treat for the
child while being closer aligned with an amount that
makes sense based on their size and body mass.

123

By following the ABCs, it gets us to *think* more consciously about sugar and its impact on our families. Below are three steps to help guide parents' *actions* when it comes to managing sugar intake in their homes. I frame this as guidance because every household and family is different, so it wouldn't be fair to assume what works for one family will always work for another. These general steps are to be used as a methodology for how to think differently about the topic of sugar—buying it and eating it. It is up to parents to figure out what is applicable and how to take the thinking and actions and extend them for their families and overall health goals.

1—If You Buy It and Store It, They'll Eat It

The best way to control sugar in your home is to not have it in your home. As we have discussed, do not keep the products in your pantry. If you buy it, you can assume someone in your house is going to consume it. Controlling diet is best managed at the grocery store. It is much easier to not buy and not have it available than it is to buy it and have it available and then try to explain to your children why they cannot have it. If you do decide to buy these items, at least keep them away from children so you can control their consumption. If you do allow these products into your home, make sure the right filters are in place so they are eaten based on a health strategy and not just because they're available.

2—Teach Good Health Habits at an Early Age

As parents we have the responsibility of teaching our children good eating habits, just as we must teach them good manners and all the other life lessons we want them to learn. Diabetes is a horrible lifelong condition that leads to blindness, amputation, and many other complications. We want our children to understand that *health matters* and is a direct outcome of what they eat and what life habits they develop. What we do today affects our health tomorrow. This life lesson will help parents not have to fight with their children about sweets. It explains the *why*.

3—Trust Common Sense, Not Commercial Advertising

Based on all of the false advertising and misinformation that has been uncovered over the last several years, it is best to just ignore and *block out* advertising altogether. Larry Olmsted did a great book on this topic entitled *Real Food Fake Food*. Below are a few examples from his findings:

Most extra virgin olive oil is fake – A study by the University of California concluded more than two-thirds of imported oils labeled "extra virgin" did not meet the legal standard and was not from extra virgin olives. The oil had been chemically modified to add taste and texture, advertised as 'extra virgin' and sold at a premium.

Most fish in sushi is mislabeled – One study found that 39% of New York restaurants and retail fish sellers sold fish that was mislabeled as did every single one of sixteen sushi restaurants tested. Boston and LA fared worse, with fake fish rates of 48% and 55% respectively. Along with this, DNA testing confirmed that one-third of 1,215 fish samples collected from 674 retail outlets in 21 states were mislabeled, according to U.S. Food and Drug Administration (FDA) guidelines.

Much of the salmon sold as wild caught is actually farmed - Asian pangasius (or ponga), a cheap farmed white fish, is frequently passed off as everything from catfish to sole to flounder to grouper and sold at a premium. Expensive red snapper is hardly ever actual red snapper and farmed fish like salmon is often sold as "wild caught."

There are so many examples of false advertising with food products it takes a whole separate book to capture. It was found, for instance, that a major bottled water company advertised being spring water and sold at a premium even though it was actually refurbished collected runoff water. Another study found that most

73

blueberry muffins do not have real blueberries. The blueberries are made from blue colored corn starch and other ingredients formed into a blue berry shape.

Many of the claims around antioxidants, vitamins and minerals, electrolytes, probiotics, etc. are not regulated or monitored by government agencies. We cannot trust the advertising on labels and have to rely on common sense. The basic rule is simple: If something comes in a container (box, carton, jar, etc.) from a manufacturing plant then the product has been manipulated. You cannot trust what is advertised accurately reflects the health benefits. If something eatable comes directly from a plant, tree or bush then it has not been manipulated (if you do not count pesticides, herbicides and GMOs). In this case you do not need to worry about or rely on the advertising to understand the health benefits. No one would ever argue whether a stalk of broccoli or tomato from the vine is healthy!

Overmarketing and advertising have become so common in our daily lives that we hardly notice or give them a second thought anymore. The strategy for companies producing most consumable goods for our children is fairly simple. Take a wheat- or corn-based product and load it with sugar or salt. Then fry or bake it. All are commodity items that get lots of federal subsidies, making them cheap to manufacture and produce. These products are then marketed, using any buzzwords the marketing department can come up with (besides sugar or salt) written in big letters on the front of the packages that sound good to parents.

For blatantly sweet products, like ice cream or candy bars, they may use *sweet* as part of the marketing strategy. But marketing departments want everyday consumables to seem healthful, so it is common to avoid using the words *sweet* and *salty* and instead get more creative. There are lots of buzzwords now, most of them irrelevant when it comes to health and fuzzy on the science. Let's take a couple of examples:

Daily supply of vitamin C: Creating a processed food or drink item and then adding ascorbic acid (the base molecular compound of vitamin C) is not the same as getting the molecules by eating food items in their natural state. An orange, for instance, has over seventy compounds that work in conjunction with vitamin C to help your body absorb and use the antioxidant productively to prevent oxidation, which is shown to cause cellular damage. Vitamin C is considered an antioxidant, which I'll talk about in a minute.

When you extract the molecular structure from the product in its natural state and add it into a processed product, there is a good chance your body is not properly absorbing the molecule or leveraging its health benefits in the most productive way. Just because a product advertises having a "daily supply of vitamin C" doesn't mean your body can or is absorbing the vitamin due to processing, making the health claim irrelevant.

Packed with a daily supply of vitamins and minerals:
Packed with vitamins and minerals usually means a lot
of added supplements and then packed with sugar and
other unhealthful ingredients. Using the supplemental
form (the molecular form of a vitamin, for instance, as
we mention above) does not mean the vitamin is being
absorbed efficiently. If you want to ensure your child is
getting the vitamins and minerals they need they should
get those from fresh fruits and vegetables. Do not rely on
processed products from a box or bottle to provide the
nutrition that a child needs to be healthy.

Packed with antioxidants: This is another abused term
manufacturers use to market children's food products to
parents. All fruits and vegetables naturally produce
antioxidants, which is just a name for molecular
compounds used to protect cells from free radical
damage. Free radicals are unstable, highly reactive forms
of oxygen or other elements or molecules, which are a
by-product of the process of making energy or doing
other tasks within a cell. Plants produce free radicals just
like we do, so we can benefit by consuming the
antioxidants in plants.

The challenge here is that molecules are most effective
in their natural state. If the fruit or vegetable is cooked or
frozen, for instance, it affects the chemistry, which
affects the molecular integrity of the antioxidant. For
example, a blueberry picked from a blueberry bush has a
lot of beneficial compounds that are good for health and
how the body works. A blueberry muffin or blueberry

granola bar (if it even has *real* blueberries) that comes off an assembly line probably has very few beneficial compounds after processing.

A broccoli floret that is picked from a broccoli plant has a lot of healthy compounds, including antioxidants. The processed broccoli florets that come in a packet in a box of chicken and broccoli pasta mix probably have virtually no antioxidant benefit. Companies will boast that their product is "packed with antioxidants" on any food that may have started as some sort of plant, even though there is probably very little health benefit because of the processing.

Be careful of all marketing. There are always new marketing terms to sell more products. The best thing is to learn to tune out the marketing jargon altogether and just buy food items in their natural state. Don't trust that the marketing accurately reflects the compromise caused by processing. You could easily buy a product whose manufacturer claims it is packed with antioxidants, even though in actuality it has little to no antioxidant benefits. Because there is very little oversight or governance on these claims and what companies can say or do in their marketing campaigns most have a sell-now-apologize-later mentality.

How much a product is compromised from a health perspective depends on the processing. Some companies are more conscious than others, but the best strategy is to always be skeptical; it is too difficult to separate fact from fiction in today's overmarketed consumer goods.

Conclusion

Having a beneficial health strategy for your family is simpler than it sounds. Navigating through the misinformation, overmarketing, and social influence to put the right filters in place in today's world—that is the hard part. It takes new levels of effort and awareness to build barriers to insulate our children from influences that work against us as parents. Keeping our children physically healthy and mentally happy requires not only protecting them from the obvious threats but also being able to identify threats that are not as obvious but compromise health. Overconsumption of sugar (one unnecessary snack at a time) is one of those not-so-obvious threats that can have devastating ramifications later in life.

Parents with small children do not want to watch them suffer with complications from type 2 diabetes in their twenties or thirties because of the poor diet and overconsumption of sugar we're allowing today. This is a real threat and requires a real response now while we have a chance to influence the outcome. I hope this book at least helps you to rethink the topic and develop a strategy that works best for your family's health goals.

Wishing health and happiness from our family to yours,

Jay

References

1. US Federal Trade Commission. *Marketing Food to Children and Adolescents: A Review of Industry Expenditures, Activities, and Self-Regulation*. Washington, DC: US Federal Trade Commission, 2008.

2. Harris, J., et al. *Sugary Drink FACTS: Evaluating Sugary Drink Nutrition and Marketing to Youth*. New Haven, CT: Rudd Center for Food Policy and Obesity, 2011.

3. "Coca-Cola: Don't Blame Us for Obesity Epidemic!" *The New York Daily News,* June 8, 2012.

4. Lesser, L. I., C. B. Ebbeling, M. Goozner, D. Wypij, and D. S. Ludwig. "Relationship between Funding Source and Conclusion among Nutrition-related Scientific Articles." *PLoS Medicine* 4 (2007): e5.

Made in the USA
Middletown, DE
09 May 2022